IØ1Ø2321

The Anchor of Our Purest Thoughts
Series

To my parents for their love and support

Praise for *Fitness Powered Brains*

"*Fitness Powered Brains* simplifies complex scientific ideas of the great benefits of exercise on our brains. It is full of practical advice that can boost your mental powers and enhance your chances for success."

— **Jean Paul Zogby**, Bestselling Author of *The Power of Time Perception*

"Chong Chen has produced a short but convincing introduction to exercise science. In simple and readable paragraphs, he conveys the many benefits of exercise, across many domains of life. Now there is no longer any excuse not to get outside and do something!"

— **Dr. Kennon M. Sheldon**, Curators' Distinguished Professor of Psychological Sciences, University of Missouri
One of 20 Most Cited Social Psychologists in the World
Former Book Review Editor for the *Journal of Positive Psychology*

"*Fitness Powered Brains* is a milestone in the field of physical fitness and brain science. Exercise was the theme of Dr. Chen's Ph.D. dissertation. As a member of the dissertation committee, I've witnessed this perfect expertise throughout his scientific career. This book is his another great achievement."

— **Dr. Masao Mizuno**, Professor of Physical Fitness Science, Hokkaido University, Japan

"An extraordinary achievement. *Fitness Powered Brains* will change how people view physical fitness and exercise. Finally we have a powerful strategy to strengthen our brains, increase our work productivity, and cope with daily stress."

— **Dr. Wei Hao**, Professor of Psychiatry,
Central South University, China
Former President, Chinese Psychiatrist Association

"We need to consider both the fitness of our body and that of our mind when searching and planning the steps that can lead us to the achievement of our personal and professional goals. Dr. Chong Chen's book provides the guidance regarding your first science-based steps toward both physical and mental fitness. Read *Fitness Powered Brains* and discover what as little as a 4 minute walk can do for your physical and psychological well-being."

— **Lucia Grosaru**, *Psychology Corner*

The Anchor of Our Purest Thoughts (Book 1)

FITNESS POWERED BRAINS

Optimize Your Productivity, Leadership and Performance

DR. CHONG CHEN

Brain & Life Publishing

London

ISBN 978-1-9997601-6-8 E-book

ISBN 978-1-9997601-7-5 Paperback

Brain & Life Publishing

27 Old Gloucester Street, London, U.K.

First Printing, 2017

For information about special needs for bulk purchases, sales promotions, and educational needs, please contact orders@brainandlife.net.

Table of Contents

FOREWORD

Do you wonder what makes some people more successful than others? Are you curious to know what secret sauce behind success is? Sure you do, and this book will give you some of the best, tested and tried, easy to implement ideas for success.

We all have a tendency to attribute many factors to success, whether it is wit, personality, wealth, or just pure chance. But behind all those factors is a common underlying denominator: Productivity and leadership come from mental fitness and that can be achieved through physical fitness.

I was intrigued with *Fitness Powered Brains* because it relates so much to my bestselling book *The Power of Time Perception*, which also covers how exercise can boost our brain's information processing speed. This always results in an experience that slows down time. Examples of great athletes with their ability to see things in "slow motion," abound from Roger Federer to Tiger Woods, and Ted Williams who once said, "I could see the laces of a baseball flying at 90 miles an hour!"

In *Fitness Powered Brains*, Dr. Chen uses the latest findings in neuroscience to confirm this same principle, mainly: how our brains and mental powers are highly boosted with regular exercise, and how this forms the key ingredient in promoting productivity, leadership, and success. Based on groundbreaking research, Dr. Chen simplifies complex scientific ideas about the great benefits of exercise on our brains. It is full of practical advice that can boost your mental powers and enhance your chances for success. These scientifically-based arguments are extremely compelling, well presented, and easy to understand. Not only that, the book covers various ways to improve emotional well-being, and sleep, work, and family related stress.

Dr. Chen's *Fitness Powered Brains* is one of the most comprehensive and authoritative books on mental excellence through physical fitness. There is so much to learn from *Fitness Powered Brains* to take into your daily life routine that will make you a better person, geared for success.

— Jean Paul Zogby, Bestselling author of
The Power of Time Perception

PREFACE

*There's no question that people who are fit
are more productive; they enjoy their work
more and accomplish more.*

— Exercise physiologist Jerome Zuckerman

The world is changing constantly, perhaps faster now than ever before, and it is up to us to keep pace with that change as we go about our daily lives. Nowhere is the pace being felt more keenly, than in the world of business. With the advent of the internet, our ability to work across the globe in the blink of an eye meant that the world contracted even more and we had to move even faster to keep up.

The demand for excellence in productivity and leadership has been two of the areas that have seen some of the greatest speeds in leaps of expectation. With that demand, new strategies are constantly being sought, to help companies and individuals to realize potential.

There are limits we encounter when working, which take something extra to overcome. But with the right approach, we can increase and expand on those limits through simply working towards making our brains more efficient and up to the challenge.

It is no secret that physically active people are more productive than those who sit around. Taking a short walk can stimulate the mind and make you more creative and happier, while even a short amount of daily exercise is a good for both physical and mental agility and can improve productivity.

This book has been written to help you understand these ideas and to assist you with achieving your own goals in life, through discovering the best ways to exercise.

The benefits of physical fitness and exercise are beginning to be realized by many. A survey of the top 3,000 U.S. companies' executives reported that two-thirds of them exercised at least three times a week. While so many busy executives are placing physical fitness and exercise at the top of their priority list, regular people have been physically inactive. In many countries, including China, Japan, the U.K., and the U.S., over 60–70% people fail to engage in the amount of exercise recommended by national and international guidelines. This suggests that the average individual's knowledge concerning the benefits of exercise is superficial, or that the willpower of regular people to maintain a physically active lifestyle is not enough.

Now is the time for you to realize the benefits of physical fitness and enhance your willpower to exercise. By being more active and fitter, you will start to enjoy a job that has perhaps become mundane, while accomplishing more at the same time.

This practical and enjoyable read is the first step towards a healthier, happier and more productive you. It is a book that has something for everyone.

PART 1: FIT PEOPLE ARE MORE EFFECTIVE

1. Fitness Predicts Success: The Lifelong Study of Harvard College Men

Physical fitness is the basis for all other forms of excellence.

— John F. Kennedy, the man from the Harvard Grant Study who later became the president of the United States

William T. Grant (1876–1972) was the founder of a chain of U.S. mass-merchandise stores bearing his name that grew to 1100 stores across the country. Grant perhaps was not the first person who wanted to find effective managers for his business, but he was definitely the first person who funded a groundbreaking study to identify what makes an effective manager. The study was the Grant Study of Adult Development at Harvard University, or more famously known as the Harvard Grant Study.

After establishing his multitude of chain stores, Grant became interested in identifying effective officers and managers for his commercial empire. Harvard was a great place to start. There, in the year 1938, Grant met the director of Harvard Health Services, Arlen V. Bock. Bock was a pioneer in the study of human physiology. It was Bock who proposed the concept of positive health.

Bock argued that instead of merely treating diseases, medical research should pay more attention to preventive measures and how to live well. Two decades later, Carl Rogers and Abraham Maslow would take this concept into the new field of humanistic psychology. Six decades after that, Martin Seligman would further extend the field into positive psychology.

Bock had been planning to establish a long-lasting study to investigate what contributes to positive health and successful living. Grant helped Bock realize this study. Grant provided the funding, and Bock organized the study. Bock assembled a team that spanned medicine, physiology, anthropology, psychiatry, psychology, and social work, and was advised by such luminaries as the physiologist Walter Cannon, psychiatrist Adolf Meyer and psychologist Henry Murray, all influential figures in the 20th century.

Bock carefully chose 268 male college students at Harvard from the sophomore classes of 1939 through 1944. He measured them from every conceivable angle and with every available scientific tool ranging from physical, psychological, familial, to social aspects. The measurement took at least 20 hours for each student. Several tests showed these men were among the top 3% of the general population in IQ (with a mean of 135) and top 5–10% of the college-bound high school graduates in Scholastic Aptitude Test scores. Furthermore, many of the men finally achieved dramatic success in their lives. Four ran for the U.S. Senate, one served in a presidential Cabinet, and one was president (John F. Kennedy). Until the year 2012, 21% of the members have been included in *Who's Who in America*, a publication containing short biographies of distinguished Americans.

The study followed the physical and emotional health and life trajectories of these men, starting with their undergraduate days, through war, career, marriage (and divorce for some), parenthood, and grandparenthood until now, who (those still alive) are in their nineties. Each year, these men had to answer hundreds of questions about many aspects of their health, marriages, families, careers, and so on. Every 10–15 years, the men were interviewed by a psychiatrist face-to-face. The study turned out to be one of the longest-running and most exhaustive studies of physical and mental well-being in history.

In 1966, psychiatrist George Vaillant became the director of the study for the next 42 years. Vaillant performed many detailed statistical analyses of the data these men provided in answering the question that Arlen

Bock asked (What factors predict positive health and successful living?) when he established the study, and the question that William Grant asked (What factors predict a good leadership and managerial success?) when he funded the study in 1938. Vaillant gathered ten achievements to form a flourishing score for each man indicating their level of success between the age of 60 to 80:

1) Included in Who's Who in America

2) Earning income in the study's top quartile

3) Low in psychological distress

4) Success and enjoyment in work, love, and play since age 65

5) Good subjective health at age 75

6) Good subjective and objective physical and mental health at age 80

7) Being actively involved in empathic nurturing of a new generation, especially adolescents and adults other than one's own children (this is based on the developmental theory of psychologist Erik Erikson, and is also vital for leadership)

8) Availability of social supports other than one's wives and kids between ages 60 and 75

9) In a good marriage between ages 60 and 80

10) Close to one's kids between ages 60 and 75

Vaillant analyzed what variables one possessed at a young age contributed to flourishing at age 60–80. He put all the data available from college up till midlife into the statistical analysis, including those physical, psychological, familial, and social data measured in college and from interviews. Vaillant found that physical fitness in college, as measured by athletic prowess and treadmill endurance, turned out to be one of the most significant factors in predicting success between the ages of 60–80. That is, those with high levels of fitness in their college years would go on to achieve greater success in their later years.

What a striking finding! People seldom think of looking at the link between fitness and success. Yet the Harvard Grant Study shows that high fitness at a young age predicts late-life success at work and home, both physically and mentally.

Why?

As we will see in later chapters, fit people have more efficient brains and create more neurons in their brains. They can also tolerate more stress. All these characteristics put them in a favorable position to achieve more. Furthermore, fitness is largely a result of regular exercise. To date, thousands of studies worldwide have provided robust evidence that exercise cultivates almost every aspect of the mental and cognitive power necessary for success at school, work, and at home.

Thus, as indicated in the Harvard Grant Study, what makes fitness so important is actually the habit of exercise. Exercise builds endurance, strength, and leads to higher levels of fitness. Those with high fitness in college tended to exercise regularly before and in college. They also exercised into their later life. It was the habit of exercise that helped them stay fit as they aged. This single habit of exercise won them a more successful life. Regular exercise was the key. It is worth noting that Arlie V. Bock, the founder of the Harvard Grant Study, himself walked two miles a day until his death at 96.

2. Fit People Have More Efficient Brains

People who say they can't find time to become fit should realize that a fitness program actually produces time.

— Dr. George Sheehan, physician, athlete, and bestselling author

Try to do this mental calculation within 10 seconds: 23 × 34.

It is easy to do it with pen and paper, but not with your mind. To do this mental calculation, you may try to multiply 23 by 30, then multiply 23 by 4, and finally add the two products together. Multiplying 23 by 30 gets you 690; multiplying 23 by 4 gets you 92; then you add 92 to…what? Did you forget the figures and have to calculate it from scratch again? It is hard.

The capacity of our brain to simultaneously hold and process multiple bits of information is called working memory. Our working memory is limited. Next time, try this experiment with your friends or family when walking together. Ask them to do this mental calculation and see whether they can keep their walking speed. There is a high probability they will stop to calculate. The mental calculation consumes all our working memory, so there is little left to control natural walking. You may also find that your mind wandering during a meeting prevents you from hearing what the speaker is saying. You see, your working memory is limited. You cannot control "two minds," one doing your own thinking, while the other is listening to people's conversations.

Working memory is one typical executive function. Executive functions represent the efficiency of our brain in processing information. Another typical executive function is cognitive flexibility, the ability to switch between thinking in different dimensions and levels, and about different concepts. One example of cognitive flexibility is flexible thinking between the big picture (e.g., forests) and the local details (e.g., trees). As popularized by the management guru Peter M. Senge at MIT, strategic management requires systems thinking, that is, solving a particular problem without damaging the system (i.e., the big picture) and inducing future problems. Systems thinking is but an expression of cognitive flexibility. Like working memory, cognitive flexibility and all other executive functions are limited. However, there does exist individual differences so some people, for instance, physically fit people (i.e., those with high endurance and strength), have higher executive functions and more efficient brains than others.

To process the same amount of information, fit people are much faster and use fewer brain resources. They are better at the above mental calculation: they can hold and process more information simultaneously. Fit people are better at reasoning and solving problems; they think more effectively and flexibly. They get things done faster, better, and with greater ease. Psychologist Charles H. Hillman at the University of Illinois at Urbana-Champaign in the U.S. reported that elementary school children with higher fitness levels, as measured by a shuttle run test, possessed executive functions higher than their peers. The fit children also were better at solving mathematical problems. Physical fitness scientist Masao Mizuno and his Ph.D. student, Toru Ishihara at Hokkaido University in Japan, made similar findings.

The observation that high fitness is associated with better executive functions holds true for adults. David Bunce at the University of London found that fit postal workers, whether young (age 18–30) or older (43–62), performed better on tasks of executive functions than other employees. Fitness improves brain efficiency and work performance. In a study done by Nicolaas P. Pronk at *HealthPartners* in the U.S., fit corporate employees finished more work than their less fit colleagues, despite devoting less effort to that same work. In another study by David Frew at Gannon University and Nealia Bruning at Kent State University, commercial real estate stock brokers who attended a 12-week-long fitness training program had higher sales during and after the program as opposed to their colleagues who did not attend. The 12-week program consisted of walking and running three times a week. Understandably, the program improved the employees' executive functions, which allowed them to think more flexibly and create more effective marketing strategies at work.

More recently, psychologists Laura Chaddock-Heyman, Arthur Kramer, and their colleagues at the University of Illinois at Urbana-Champaign used the technique of functional magnetic resonance imaging (FMRI) to study the brain activities of children who underwent a fitness training program. FMRI measures brain activity by detecting changes associated with blood flow. It relies on the observation that when the activity of a brain area is increased, blood flow to that region also increases. In this study, Chaddock-Heyman, Kramer, and their colleagues asked 7–9 year old children to exercise for two hours each day after school for nine months. They found this exercise program improved the children's endurance (running on a treadmill with increasing speed until volitional exhaustion) by 6%. Meanwhile, the program improved these children's executive function. Compared to brain activation before the program, these children's brain activation in the right prefrontal cortex during an executive function task exhibited a decrease following the program. The prefrontal cortex is the CEO of our brain. This reduced activation in the right prefrontal cortex reflects the greater efficiency of the brain in achieving effective performance. On similar tasks, people with higher IQs generally show lower (more efficient) brain activity in the prefrontal cortex. Chaddock-Heyman, Kramer, and their colleagues found that, after 9 months of exercise, these children showed similar performance and brain patterns as a group of 22-year old sedentary young adults. Stated differently, the 9-month-long two hours of daily exercise improved these children's executive functions by 13–15 years. Remarkable. Fitness training considerably improves brain efficiency.

The great news is that fitness training improves brain efficiency not only in children but also in adults and aged people. After reviewing 18 experimental studies in adults and aged people, Arthur Kramer and his colleague, Stanley Colcombe concluded that fitness training improves executive functions, with a long-term of training being the most effective.

Fitness provides individuals with one of the most powerful strategies to improve performance: more efficient brains. Fit people can solve problems faster, better, and easier. The argument by physician, athlete, and bestselling author Dr. George Sheehan captures this point: "People who say they can't find time to become fit should realize that a fitness program actually produces time."

3. Fit People Create More Neurons in Their Brains

Those who cannot remember the past are condemned to repeat it.

— George Santayana, *Reason in Common Sense*, Volume 1 of *The Life of Reason* (1905)

A recent breakthrough made in neuroscience and psychology was the discovery of the capacity of the adult brain to regenerate neurons, i.e., adult neurogenesis. The number of new neurons dramatically affects people's ability to memorize new information. It is exciting to note that the number of new neurons in the brains of fit individuals far surpasses those in the brains of less fit people. More neurons provide fit individuals with the robust neural substrate to memorize more information.

Throughout the vast majority of the twentieth century, leading neuroscientists considered the nervous system incapable of regeneration. It was believed that we are born with all our neurons, and no neurons can be produced after birth. Neurons only die and cannot be renewed. However, American biologist Joseph Altman proved that neurons continue to be generated in the adult rat brain, particularly in an area called the dentate gyrus in the hippocampus. The hippocampus is famous for its critical role in forming episodic memory, in transforming short-term memory into long-term memory, and in spatial navigation. In 1998, Fred Gage at the Salk Institute for Biological Studies in La Jolla, California showed that the human brain, specifically the dentate gyrus of the hippocampus, produces new neurons even in adulthood. It has now been estimated that approximately 6% of the total number of neurons are generated each month in the dentate gyrus. The newborn neurons are required for behavioral pattern separation, a process that transforms similar experiences into distinct and non-overlapping memory representations. Newborn neurons separately encode new memory while keeping the old memory stored in the old neurons undisturbed. These newborn neurons make our memory more accurate.

In humans, the cerebral blood volume (CBV) and cerebral blood flow (CBF) in the hippocampus, especially in the dentate gyrus, have been markers of the amount of adult neurogenesis. This is based on the observation that neurogenesis occurs within an angiogenic niche; most of the dividing cells are at the growing terminus of small capillaries. More neurogenesis is associated with more capillaries. The increase in capillaries induces an increase in CBV and CBF, which can be easily assayed in humans with perfusion techniques. Recently, it has been reported that endurance (namely aerobic fitness, see Chapter 5) is positively associated with the hippocampal CBF. Individuals with higher levels of aerobic fitness show higher levels of hippocampal CBF, which suggests that they create more neurons in their brains. This increased number of neurons gains them an enhanced ability to memorize new information.

The ability to memorize new information is fundamental for humans. The consequences of the accumulation of memory are one's stored knowledge, namely crystallized intelligence and wisdom. Higher crystallized intelligence and wisdom definitely benefits work performance and leadership skills. Fitness earns people more neurons and places them in an advantageous position to gain more crystallized intelligence and wisdom.

The team of Fred Gage, the discoverer of adult human neurogenesis, reported that a 12-week aerobic fitness training program increased participants' new neurons in the brain. In this study, 21–45 year old subjects performed one-hour-long exercise which included cycling, treadmill running, climbing, and so on four times a week. It was found that the 12 weeks of exercise increased dentate gyrus CBV, the marker of neurogenesis. Furthermore, the increase in CBV was correlated with a subject's performance in a later memory test. This suggests that aerobic fitness training promotes neurogenesis and improves memory. It is consistent with findings from animal experiments performed by Gage's team that mice raised in cages with a running wheel created 54% more new neurons in 12 days than those raised in cages without a running wheel. The mice raised in cages with a running wheel also exhibited superior spatial memory compared to those without.

Besides, Gage's team also noticed another interesting phenomenon. The increased dentate gyrus CBV after the 12-week exercise program correlated with subjects' aerobic fitness levels at baseline. The more fit at baseline, the more increased dentate gyrus CBV after the program. That is, fitter individuals created more neurons after the same training. They benefited more from the same amount of exercise. This is like the Matthew effect in economics and sociology that "the rich get richer and the poor get poorer." Aerobic fitness is like private capital. High aerobic fitness gains people an accumulated advantage to benefit more from future exercise. The more you exercise, the more fit you become, the more benefit you get out of it.

4. Fit People Have Higher Stress Tolerance

The healthier and stronger I am, the more relaxed I am, the better it is for the company.

— Richard E. Snyder, former Chairman and CEO of Simon & Schuster Publishing

A certain level of stress is helpful. If nothing in your work is challenging, you are in your safe zone. You will never reach your full potential and maximize your performance. Without challenges and the stress that comes with it, you will never get stronger, let alone achieve what Abraham Maslow called self-actualization. As a leader, you can always lower your fiscal year goals to reduce your and your employees' stress, but your organization will never grow. A certain level of stress motivates you to work harder and achieve more.

However, too much stress becomes detrimental. If you set your fiscal year goals too high, you and your employees will suffer from lots of pressure. Excessive stress from work is bad for your health, both mentally and physically. Numerous neuroscientific studies have shown that excessive stress reduces brain efficiency and the number of new neurons in the brain. It impairs people's executive functions and memory. When excessive stress is prolonged, people may eventually

24

develop a syndrome called "burnout," becoming emotionally exhausted, desperate, indifferent to other people, and doubt their own abilities. Physically, they experience fatigue, pain, and other psychosomatic symptoms. Executive burnout has unfortunately become very widespread; we will touch upon this in Chapter 8. Stressed people show reduced work performance and often lower their goals to reduce stress. Their final achievement is severely compromised.

For every individual, there is a certain threshold for stress. When the level of stress is below this threshold, people feel safe, comfortable, and motivated. When the level of stress is above this threshold, people feel nervous, sad, angry, get insomnia, and easily give up. This threshold, the amount of stress people can handle without getting overwhelmed, is called stress tolerance. Just as it is far more effective and less expensive to prevent than to treat many physical diseases, it is far more effective and less expensive to prevent than to treat stress related problems. A practical and important task for modern psychology and medicine is to find effective strategies to increase this threshold for people. Recently psychology and medicine found one preventive measure: fitness and exercise. Individuals with higher fitness levels and people who exercise regularly have increased stress tolerance. Their threshold for stress is higher. Given the same stress, these people show reduced physiological and psychological responses. They are psychologically stronger. Below I will give you two typical examples of laboratory stress which fit people and people who exercise regularly show high tolerance.

Suppose as a volunteer you are in the laboratory of a psychology department. You are involved in two experiments. The first experiment starts. You are asked to immerse your left hand into a basin of icy water for 60 seconds. You put your left hand into the water: it is cold! You feel pain in your hand and want to get your hand out of the icy water as soon as possible. But you recall that the experiment lasts for only 60 seconds and it is no more than a single, painful experience; you hang on until the end.

After two to three hours of rest, you are at the second experiment. You are asked to give a 5-minute speech introducing yourself. In front of you are two well-dressed interviewers, seated upright with stoic facial expressions. You are puzzled and wondering what to say about yourself. While giving the speech, you occasionally hear one interviewer say, "You are slow," and "Come on, hurry up." You get nervous, but you finish the speech, and are asked to perform a 5-minute mental arithmetic test before these two interviewers. Your task is to subtract seven from any number they give you serially before it gets to the minus. But it seems no matter how fast you calculate, one interviewer always tells you to "go faster." It is tough.

These two procedures are typical stressors used by psychologists in the laboratory. The first one is a physical stressor, while the second one is a social stressor. Both have been found to induce robust physiological and psychological stress responses in subjects. For instance, in response to these stressors, physiologically people show increases in blood pressure, heart rate, levels of body arousal (as shown by skin conductance), and the stress hormone cortisol. Psychologically, people report increases in nervousness, sadness, and even anger.

Interestingly, when subjected to this kind of stressor, people who perform better on the shuttle run test, which measures aerobic fitness, show less physiological and psychological responses than those who perform poorly. They exhibit much less increase in blood pressure, heart rate, arousal, and cortisol levels. They also report less increase in nervousness, sadness, and anger. Similarly, people who exercise regularly, even merely once per week, show less physiological and psychological responses compared to those who don't.

Fitness and regular exercise raise people's threshold for stress. Fit people and those who regularly exercise can tolerate more stress. This means they can set higher goals and reach their fullest potential more often. As they also have more efficient brains and a greater number of new neurons in the brain, they have a far better chance to achieve more.

PART 2: HOW TO BUILD FITNESS

5. A Primer on Fitness: Fundamental Recommendations

With regular exercise programs, the gains we see in VO2 max (i.e., aerobic capacity) between the old and young are similar.

— Dr. William J. Evans, director of the Noll Laboratory for Human Performance Research at Pennsylvania State University

Two keys for building optimal fitness are regular exercise and a healthy diet.

Without exercise, fitness drops about 30–50% from age 30 to 80. Exercise can minimize this drop. Exercise takes two forms: aerobic and resistance. I have been asked and often puzzled by the question (and for a long time): Which is more beneficial for humans, aerobic or resistance exercise? This is a fundamental question.

Aerobic exercise, also known as endurance activity or cardiovascular exercise, involves a sustained period of rhythmic movement of large muscles. It requires the pumping of oxygenated blood by the heart to deliver oxygen to the muscles to generate energy. Examples of aerobic exercise include walking, jogging, running, cycling, swimming, dancing, playing soccer, basketball, tennis, and more. Aerobic fitness is typically evaluated by the one-mile walking test, the PACER test, or a treadmill running test. The one-mile walking test is perhaps the easiest to perform. In this test, you must walk as fast as you can for one mile. "Walk" means one foot must always be on the ground. The time (in minutes and seconds) you take to finish reflects your aerobic fitness. Note that a 3–5 minute warmup (stretching and brisk walking) before and cooldown (slow walk) following the test is recommended.

Resistance exercise, or anaerobic exercise, is brief, short-lasting muscle-strengthening activities, such as sprinting, jumping, weightlifting, pushups, and sit-ups. It involves major muscle groups of the legs, hips, back, abdomen, chest, shoulders, and arms. Fitness evaluated by resistance exercise is called muscle strength. An easy way to test your muscle strength is doing as many pushups or sit-ups as you can within 60 seconds. The former targets the muscles of the chest, arms, and shoulders, while the latter targets the abdominals.

As we mentioned earlier in this book, a survey of the top 3,000 U.S. companies' executives reported that two-thirds of the executives exercised at least three times weekly. Over 90% of the executives use aerobic exercise as their main workout. Is aerobic exercise more beneficial? Is resistance exercise a waste of time?

Regarding benefits on executive functions and memory, aerobic exercise is better than resistance exercise. In contrast, regarding benefits on relieving stress and regulating mood, resistance exercise is better than aerobic exercise. Moreover, several recent studies suggest that aerobic and resistance exercise may have different influences on neurotrophic factors. Whereas aerobic exercise increases serum levels of brain-derived neurotrophic factor (BDNF), resistance exercise increases serum level of insulin-like growth factor 1 (IGF-1). Both BDNF and IGF-1 are members of the neurotrophin family of growth factors which support the production, growth, differentiation, and survival of neurons. Thus, aerobic and resistance exercise may benefit the brain through different molecular mechanisms. Combined training of aerobic and resistance exercise will have the largest impact on the brain and mind. So we need not worry too much about which kind of exercise brings the biggest benefits. Do both.

The next question I often hear is: How much exercise is necessary to build fitness? Dozens of studies have found that the amount of exercise recommended by various national and international guidelines is robustly effective in building fitness. Here is the recommended amount for adults by the WHO: Throughout the week, do at least 150 minutes of moderate-intensity aerobic exercise, or at least 75 minutes of vigorous-intensity aerobic exercise, or an equivalent combination of both.

While doing moderate-intensity exercise, you should be able to talk but not sing. Typical examples of moderate-intensity aerobic exercises are brisk walking, double tennis, table tennis, gardening, and ballroom dancing. While doing vigorous-intensity exercise, you cannot talk without pausing for breath. Typical examples of vigorous-intensity aerobic exercise are jogging, single tennis, swimming laps, and jumping rope.

For resistance exercise, do at least 20 minutes of resistance exercise three times a week.

Engaging in the above amount of aerobic and resistance exercise might be challenging at first, but recall what Dr. George Sheehan said: "People who say they can't find time to become fit should realize that a fitness program actually produces time."

The second key to fitness is a healthy diet. High saturated fat diet (such as butter, cheese, fatty beef) and overweight/obesity (namely BMI or weight in kilograms divided by the square of height in meters >=25) are the enemies of fitness, executive functions, memory, and health. Both reduce the number of new neurons in the brain. I have written a chapter on how to lose weight in another book *Plato's Insight: How Physical Exercise Boosts Mental Excellence*. Feel free to check it out. To summarize briefly, if you are overweight or obese, a good first step is to reduce your energy intake by 500–750 kcal per day, stick to a Mediterranean-style diet, and exercise.

1) The Mediterranean-style diet refers to the traditional dietary practices of countries bordering the Mediterranean Sea. It is characterized by:

2) High consumption of plant foods: vegetables, fruits, legumes, and cereals

3) High intake of olive oil as the principal source of monounsaturated fat, but low intake of saturated fat such as butter, cheese, and fatty beef

4) Moderate intake of fish

5) Low to moderate intake of dairy products

6) Low consumption of meat and poultry

7) Wine consumed in low to moderate amounts

Studies involving millions of people have consistently reported that high adherence to the Mediterranean-style diet is associated with healthier body weight, better cognitive functions, and better overall health.

Regular exercise and a healthy diet are highly effective in improving the fitness of millions of people. They should also be effective for you. Give it a try.

PART 3: CREATIVE USE OF EXERCISE TO BOOST PERFORMANCE

6. Taking a Walk Leads to More Creativity than Sitting

Physical fitness is a pre-requisite for creativity.

— Japanese novelist Haruki Murakami, *What I Talk About When I Talk About Running* (2007)

The Japanese novelist Haruki Murakami is a runner. He jogs 10 km every day, because Murakami believes jogging is important for his novelist career. It gains him not only strength, but also a certain liberty of the mind. In *What I Talk About When I Talk About Running*, Murakami writes that he jogs to gain a state of mental blank, during which random thoughts come. These random thoughts might sometimes turn into a creative idea. Exercise promotes creativity.

The best example supporting this argument is from Charles Darwin. As written in his autobiography, Darwin walked routinely along the "sandwalk" near his home. This habit was not just for his physical health. It was a pivotal part of his intellectual routine. During walking, many of his puzzles were solved. Darwin called the "sandwalk" his "thinking path." Recently, Michael Mangum, the president and CEO of the Mangum Group, said something similar,

"I do believe fitness impacts my job. I usually exercise during the middle of the day, say, one to four PM or so. I find that my energy is much enhanced when I return from a workout. Further, I find that because I choose to go during the day, my thoughts tend toward work while exercising. I have some of my most creative thought when working out."

The possibility that the process of exercising itself may generate creative ideas has been subjected to a scientific test. Two psychologists at Stanford University, Marily Oppezzo and Daniel Schwartz asked subjects to think of as many as possible alternate uses of an item within four minutes. People's performance on this test has been found to reflect their creativity in everyday life and at work. One example in this test was upon hearing "button," one subject thought of "as a doorknob for a dollhouse, an eye for a doll, a tiny strainer, to drop behind you to keep your path." Oppezzo and Schwartz found that participants on average thought of six novel alternate uses for one set of tests while seated in a small room facing a blank wall. Surprisingly, they thought of ten novel uses for another set of tests while walking at a comfortable pace on a treadmill facing the same wall. It suggests that people are more creative during walking compared to being seated. This observation was confirmed using another creativity test of the ability to think of original analogies to capture complex ideas. Given "light bulb blowing out," one may think of "throwing up while you are drinking." Given "budding cocoon," one may think of "coming out of a meditation retreat." Oppezzo and Schwartz found that, compared to being seated, people think of better analogies when walking on a treadmill and this beneficial effect lasts even after the walking episode.

In a later experiment, Oppezzo and Schwartz asked subjects to perform these two tests either in a sit-sit condition or a walking-sit condition. That is, in the first session, subjects performed the tests while sitting or walking on a treadmill, and in the second session, all performed the tests while sitting. Oppezzo and Schwartz found that after walking during the first session, subjects performed much worse when they sat for the second session. However, they did perform better than those who sat for both sessions. It suggests that the beneficial effect of walking on creativity lasts even when the walking has finished and that even a brief walking (i.e., four minutes) works.

Actually, Oppezzo and Schwartz were not the first to discover that exercise boosts creativity. Two decades ago, Hannah Steinberg at Middlesex University had investigated whether aerobic exercise improves people's subsequent creative thinking. Steinberg asked subjects to think of as many as possible alternate uses for tin can, either after 25 minutes of aerobic workout or after watching a 25-minute long neutral documentary video of rock formations. Steinberg found those after an aerobic workout could think of more diverse responses compared to those that watched the video. However, that was not all the experiment revealed. Steinberg asked the subjects to return to the laboratory the next day. Those who did the aerobic workout the previous day were now asked to watch the 25-minute long video, while those who watched the video the previous day were now asked to do 25 minutes of aerobic dance. After this manipulation, all subjects were asked to take the creative thinking test again, but this time, they have to think of as many as possible alternate uses for a new item, cardboard box. This time, it was those who danced for 25 minutes that thought of more diverse responses. Together these two days of experiments suggest that aerobic exercise promotes subsequent creative thinking.

From these personal experiences and psychological studies, we can glean two pieces of take-home message. First, the random ideas that come to you when exercising are not at all random. Some are often creative.

Give them a second thought and see whether they help you in a novel way. Second, even brief periods of exercise, such as four minutes of walking promotes later creative thinking, and you can take advantage of this benefit. For instance, brief walks or other forms of aerobic exercise before an interview or a meeting which requires innovation and creativity should be helpful (so long as it doesn't tire you beforehand).

7. Exercise is the Most Effective Strategy to Deal with a Bad Day

A CEO's role is probably the loneliest in the business. They're expected to be always on their game. They're not allowed to have a bad day.

— A managing director

A certain level of stress is helpful and necessary to maximize performance. But sometimes stress may outrage. Consequently, we must cope with stress before it gets out of control and causes burnout.

Many work experiences are stressful: deadlines, dealing with difficult employees, putting on a happy face before customers, being scolded by superiors, aborted projects, merging with other companies, going through reorganizations, losing contracts, reduced sales, failed products. When people feel stressed, they experience negative moods. They become dissatisfied with the job, feel fatigued, sad, and anxious, and lose interest in things or activities that they previously enjoyed. So here comes the question: What is the most effective strategy to regulate these negative moods?

More than two decades ago, psychologist Robert Thayer at California State University asked people to report the most effective and successful strategies they used to deal with a bad day. Interestingly, most people listed exercise as the number one most effective strategy. Here is the ranking of the most effective strategies based on people's answers.

1) Exercise

2) Listening to music

3) Calling, talking to or being with someone

4) Tending to chores

5) Resting, napping or sleeping

6) Using cognitive regulation strategies such as controlling thoughts, checking or analyzing the situation, or putting feelings in perspective

7) Avoiding the thing/person causing the mood

8) Being alone

The conclusion that exercise is the most effective strategy in regulating bad mood is supported by a recent study done by Maxime Taquet at Harvard Medical School. Over an approximately 4-week long period, Taquet asked over 28,000 people to report their real-time mood and activities they had been engaging through a multiplatform smartphone application. Taquet found that, when people felt bad, they played sports most often. Following sports were nature, leisure, chatting, culture, drinking, playing, and eating. More importantly, doing sports produced the most significant mood enhancement compared to the other activities. The ranking of the most effective strategies people used is shown here:

1) Sport

2) Nature

3) Culture

4) Leisure

5) Chatting

6) Drinking

7) Playing

8) Eating

Exercise is the most effective strategy to deal with a bad day.

A second question is this: How much exercise is required to enhance one's mood and reduce stress? Robert Thayer found that brisk walking for only ten minutes is enough to decrease the feeling of tension and perceived seriousness of various personal problems. It is also sufficient to increase energy and optimism. Some effects may last for as long as two hours after walking.

When stressed, many people eat sugary snacks (comfort food), smoke, or drink to cope. These coping strategies do, in the short term, change people's perception of stress and problems and reduce negative moods. However, eventually, they become detrimental to the body and brain and reduce people's problem-solving ability. An old Chinese saying goes like this: *yinzhenzhike*, which means quenching a thirst with poison. Consuming junk food, smoking, and drinking to cope with stress are typical examples of *yinzhenzhike*.

Thayer found that walking briskly for ten minutes is more effective in improving energy and lowering tension over eating a candy bar. Also, walking for five minutes before smoking a cigarette or eating a sugary snack considerably reduces the urge to smoke or snack and lengthens the time until the next cigarette is smoked or snack is eaten. It suggests that exercise can be a substitute for smoking or snacking to enhance mood and reduce stress. Not only walking, any exercise or sport is effective in enhancing one's mood. Hundreds of studies have proved that one single session of exercise, be it cycling, running, jogging, swimming, dancing, or yoga is associated with a decrease in perceived stress, fatigue, anxiety, depression, and an increase in energy and vigor. These observations provide robust evidence supporting exercise as a powerful strategy to reduce stress and regulate mood.

So next time you are having a bad day, exercise to recharge yourself. When you have to talk problems over with your employees or superiors, ask them to go out for a walk or workout together. You can talk about the problem either during or after the walking or workout. It reduces your employees' and superiors' tension and perceived stress, as well as your own. A win-win situation.

8. Exercise for Executives Burnout

Managers tend to rely on their best people; but the best people are more vulnerable to becoming burned-out people.

— Harry Levinson, When Executives Burn Out.
Harvard Business Review (1981)

What is burnout? Burnout occurs when you have lots of pressure or burdens. You put in lots of effort to achieve something or solve a problem, but you don't achieve anything. You work days, nights, and weekends for months, but you feel trapped. The result has been promising, but attaining it seems impossible. You feel tired, sad, helpless, desperate, and angry. You have headaches and difficulty falling asleep at night. You become easily offended, express suspicions towards people, and care less about people's feelings. You also feel guilty, because you have devoted all this effort to work, sacrificing the time you wanted to spend with your family. Eventually, you begin to doubt yourself about your abilities. You feel lost. You start to question your purpose of living. You are suffering from burnout.

Burnout has been around for a while. Several large-scale surveys have estimated that roughly 30% of teachers and corporate employees suffer from prolonged burnout. Burnout in executives is more severe, as managerial jobs involve contact with other people at different hierarchies and are especially demanding. In one study performed by researchers at Harvard Medical School, 96% of senior leaders reported being burned out to some degree with one-third describing their burnout as extreme. As Dr. Srini Pillay at Harvard Medical School has put, "High-functioning people actually are able to power through, but they do eventually crash."

People with prolonged burnout perform poorly on tests of executive function and memory. They also show more frequent cognitive failures in daily life. They are more likely to forget appointments and where they have put things, and are more likely to be involved in car accidents. Meanwhile, their capacity for empathy towards other people, standing in other people's perspective and showing consideration towards other people, grows impaired. Psychiatrist Hidehiko Takahashi at Kyoto University found that when watching other people's hands being harmed by a knife, hammer, or icepick, people with high burnout exhibited reduced activations in brain regions related to empathy. This reduced empathy impairs people's ability to deal with interpersonal relationships, which is at the core of "people-work" and managerial jobs. All these characteristics exhibited by burned out executives further reduced their capacity to address the situation they have been put in and trap them in a vicious cycle.

For burned out executives, the priority is to manage your burnout before it causes more damage. At this moment, rather than struggling with yourself at work, all you have to do is take a good rest and recharge yourself. The benefits of returning refreshed after pausing and recharging are worth the time away and often lead to greater creativity and less stress. Unfortunately however, 72% of executives, according to a 2015 survey by the Creative Staffing Group, won't take days off for vacations even if their company initiated an unlimited vacation policy.

When I was a graduate student at Hokkaido University, there was a course called *Society and Health* held by physical fitness scientist Masao Mizuno, health scientist Akito Kawaguchi, and hot spring scientist Yoshinori Ohtsuka (who has published *Hot Spring Therapy: Approach to Healing* (2001) and *New Hot Spring Therapy* (2012), both in Japanese and translated into Chinese). They lectured on how people can improve their health through exercise/sports, healthy diet, and spending time in nature/resorts. I personally think that a combination of exercise, healthy diet (see Chapter 5 for the recommended Mediterranean-style diet), and time spent in nature are the best combination of strategies to create positive health. Here, for the management of burnout, a combination of these three strategies is particularly effective. I focus below on the therapeutic effects of exercise on burnout.

Magnus Lindwall at the University of Gothenburg, Sweden, performed a six-year-long follow-up study of over 3,700 health care and social insurance workers. He found that, whereas those who had more exercise showed less burnout at baseline, those who increased exercise across the six-year period showed reduced burnout six years later. Here exercise ranged from gardening, walking, bicycling, dancing, swimming, to playing soccer, and so on. The correlation coefficient between increased exercise and reduced burnout was 0.79, which means that increased exercise accounts for 62.4% of the reduced burnout. In a meta-analysis (a statistical technique for integrating findings from multiple studies) of 70 interventional studies involving over 6,800 subjects, Timothy Puetz at the University of Georgia found that as short as 4–6 weeks of exercise intervention is effective in increasing energy, vigor, and decreasing burnout and fatigue. Interestingly, Puetz also found that the benefits of strength training are greater than aerobic exercise.

So give yourself a break. After recharging, you will have a brand-new view of your world and your previous problems.

A final word: Prevention is the best cure. Establish a habit of exercise. As estimated by a recent report, exercising for at least 150 minutes per week at moderate-intensity or 75 minutes at vigorous intensity reduces the risk of burnout by 62%.

9. Exercise for Work-Family Conflict

One can live magnificently in this world, if one knows how to work and how to love, to work for the person one loves and to love one's work.

— Leo Tolstoy, letter to his fiancé
Valeria Arsenev (1856)

For most people, there has always been work-family conflict. Time is limited. More time at work means less time with family and children. Worse, people do not simply go back home after work: they go back home tired and stressed. Additionally, many people are experiencing family stress, such as marital conflict and child-rearing stress, and they may bring stress to work from home. These two phenomena have been termed "work-family conflict" or "work-family spillover".

Work-family conflict hurts both job performance and family. The observation that family stress is one major source of life stress and impairs workplace performance is well known. Those with more work-family conflict do poorly at work. That work-family conflict also hurts family has been recently reported. In many industries, people have to put on a happy face at work, which is known as "surface acting." In one study by Morgan Krannitz at The Pennsylvania State

University, the more often hotel managers engage in surface acting at work, the more emotionally exhausted and anxious they feel. As a result, their partners report more work-family conflict and are more likely to want them to quit the job. Tired hotel managers are poor at controlling their emotions and devoting effort to activities at home. In another study of male employees of multinational corporations and their wives, Dutch psychologist Josje Dikkers at Radboud University Nijmegen found that when husbands reported higher workload and more psychological health complaints, their wives (whether working or not) experienced higher home load. A day's work consumes the husbands' cognitive and physical resources. After work and back at home, it becomes difficult for these tired husbands to help their wives with household duties.

Dual-earner couples are increasing, which reinforces the work-family conflict. Work-family conflict hurts not only one's partner but also the child. Children in families with more work-family conflict report worse quality of relationship with their parents. A warm parent-child relationship is a fundamental base for the child to explore the outside world and develop him- or herself. Recall the Harvard Grant Study we introduced in Chapter 1. The study followed 268 Harvard college men throughout their career, marriage, parenthood and grandparenthood. We mentioned those with high levels of fitness at college achieved more both at work and home in their later life. A warm childhood (as reported at college and in an interview with their mothers) is another significant factor. Those with a warmer childhood were more likely to achieve success and enjoy their work and life. Work-family conflict ultimately hurts the future of one's child. These negative outcomes induced by work-family conflict eventually bring more problems. Another vicious circle.

It is crucial for people to realize the existence of this vicious circle and use effective strategies to prevent and solve work-family conflict. Even if tired from work, you have to use your empathic concern, perspective taking, and effective communication skills at home. You have to carefully and considerately interact with your family. This is hard, but practice makes perfect. One way to facilitate this practice is first to recharge yourself, relieve your stress and tiredness, and increase your work efficiency through exercise.

Given the benefit of exercise on relieving stress and boosting physical, mental and cognitive power and creative thinking, people who regularly exercise have less work-family conflict and are less affected by work-family conflict. In 2007, Eva Roos at the University of

Helsinki, Finland, surveyed over 5,000 employees and found those who regularly take part in exercise report less work-family conflict. More recently in 2015, in a nine-year-long national survey of middle-aged employees, David M. Almeida at The Pennsylvania State University found that an increase in negative work-family spillover across the nine-year period was associated with decreased physical health and increased number of chronic conditions. However, more time spent on leisure time exercise buffered this association so for employees who regularly exercised during their leisure time, the increase in negative work-family spillover was only weakly associated with decreased physical health and increased number of chronic conditions nine years later.

In another book, *Plato's Insight: How Physical Exercise Boosts Mental Excellence*, I wrote, "Exercise with your child. It raises your child's IQ and self-regulation as well as your own. A win-win situation." In that book, I introduced evidence showing that children who exercised with their parents show more physical, cognitive and mental benefits than those who exercised alone or with their friends. Exercise as a family helps to solve work-family conflict and provides three degrees of benefit: to the husband, the wife, and the child.

10. Exercise Increases Positive Emotions

Self-actualizing people, that is, psychologically healthy, psychologically 'superior' people are better cognizers and perceivers. This may be true even at the sensory level itself; for example, it would not surprise me if they turned out to be more acute about differentiating fine hue differences, etc.

— Abraham Maslow, The Farther Reaches of Human Nature (1993)

People in the managerial world are not unfamiliar with terms like positivity. Abraham Maslow's concept of self-actualization and hierarchy of needs have been popular for a while. The humanistic psychology established by Maslow more than half a century ago was extended into positive psychology by Martin Seligman in the late 1990s. A major focus of positive psychology is positive emotions, including joy, gratitude, serenity, interest, hope, pride, amusement, inspiration, and love. In daily life, it is true that achievement increases our positive emotions; it is also true that positive emotions make us achieve more. Here, I will give you two examples of the benefit of positive emotions.

First, positive emotions not only feel good, but also increase people's creative thoughts. When asked to perform various cognitive tasks, people with positive emotions show more creativity and cognitive flexibility than those with neutral emotions. In a frequently used candle task, subjects are presented with a box of tacks, a candle, and a book of matches. The subjects are asked to attach the candle to the wall (a corkboard) in such a way it will burn without dripping wax on the table or floor. The difficulty of this problem arises from the functional fixedness of the box, which contains thumb-tacks. It is a container in the problem situation but must be used as a shelf in the solution situation. Psychologists found that inducing positive emotions improves subjects' performance on this task. Under positive emotional influence, subjects could more easily go beyond the routine functional fixedness view of the box and creatively use it as a shelf.

That positive emotion promotes creativity has also been observed in real life. Harvard management scientist Teresa Amabile once asked company employees to keep a journal of their everyday moods. She also asked team leaders and team members to evaluate creative thinking and work performance demonstrated by these employees. Amabile found that positive moods on the previous day predicted employees' creative thinking and performance. The more the positive moods on the previous day, the more the employees developed creative ideas and the higher their performance. Furthermore, the more the negative moods, the less creative ideas and lower the performance.

Second, positive emotions build interpersonal resources. People who experience and express positive emotions more often have more relational resources. They are more socially connected and show higher life satisfaction. The most typical expression of positive emotions is smiling. Neuroscientific research has shown that viewing smiling faces activates almost the same neural reward circuitry as monetary reward, images of one's romantic partner or child, attractive faces, aesthetic stimuli (either natural or artistic: classic art, impressionist art, landscapes, and urban scenes), humor, and pleasurable music excerpts. The same regions also activate when people think that others like, understand, or want to meet them.

Positive psychologists have identified many positive strategies to boost positive emotions. You may want to refer to these books for an extensive discussion of those strategies.

Martin Seligman, *Authentic Happiness* (2002); *Flourish: A Visionary New Understanding of Happiness and Well-being* (2011)

Tal Ben-Shahar, *Happier: Learn the Secrets to Daily Joy and Lasting Fulfillment* (2007); *Even Happier: A Gratitude Journal for Daily Joy and Lasting Fulfillment* (2010)

Here, we introduce exercise as another powerful strategy. Earlier we have shown that exercise is the most effective strategy to regulate negative moods. It is also effective in increasing positive moods.

In her master's thesis at Yoshinori Ohtsuka's lab at Hokkaido University, my friend Lili Yue studied the therapeutic effect of forest bathing (saunter in the woods). She found several walking trails perfect for forest bathing on our campus (Hokkaido University Sapporo Campus). Our campus is covered with woods, rivers, ponds, and farms. It is really beautiful and suitable for forest bathing in early summer, at which time Lili did her research. She asked college students to walk along the walking trails she specified. Lili then did a series of physiological and questionnaire measurements before and after the walk. One interesting result she found was the students showed improved positive moods after walking for 30 minutes. After walking, the students were full of energy and felt refreshed. In this case, both exercise and the natural environment (forest) contributed to their improved moods.

Even brief exercise promotes a positive mood. More than three decades ago, Robert Thayer at California State University found that brisk walking for only 5–10 minutes is enough to increase energy and optimism. More recently, Cheryl J. Hansen at Northern Arizona University found that cycling at moderate-intensity (people are able to talk, but unable to sing) improved vigor after 10 minutes following the start of the cycling, which was further enhanced after 20 and 30 minutes.

These findings provide further support for using exercise to boost creativity, work performance, and interpersonal relationships.

11. Exercise Makes You Sleep Soundly

If sleep does not serve an absolutely vital function, then it is the biggest mistake the evolutionary process ever made.

— Allan Rechtschaffen & Anthony Kales, *A Manual of Standardized Terminology Techniques and Scoring System for Sleep Stages of Human Subjects* (1968)

In 1999, Yvonne Harrision and James Horne, two professors at Loughborough University in the U.K., developed a computer game of marketing. They then found a group of MBA students to play the game. Just as they would in their future careers, each student was asked to promote sales of a product to achieve max profitability. Unknown to them, the dynamics of the marketplace changed halfway through the game when more competitors joined to sell similar products. Suddenly, strategies that previously worked failed them. Only students who recognized that they needed to change their strategy survived. Harrison and Horne split the students into two groups. Those in the first group slept as much as they wished while those in the second had their sleep deprived for 36 hours. Students who slept watched their sales suffer when new competitors first entered, but most changed their strategy and recovered quickly. In contrast, the sleep-deprived students could not cope with the unseen changes in the game. They continued to rely on what had worked before, not recognizing that the environment has changed and soon went bankrupt.

Enough sleep is required for effective decision-making. When deprived of sleep, the brain fails to react to the changing environment. In a 2010 meta-analysis of 70 laboratory studies, Julian Lim and David Dinges at the University of Pennsylvania found that 24–48 hours of sleep deprivation have a deleterious effect on every aspect of executive function and short-term memory. After staying awake without sleeping for a consecutive 24 to 48 hours, subjects fail to accurately detect visual or auditory stimuli on a computer screen, keep them in working memory, and recall them several minutes and hours later. Given the detrimental effect of sleep deprivation on the brain and mind, no wonder the above MBA students in Harrison and Horne's experiment failed to adapt their marketing strategy in response to the changed environment.

Compared to the laboratory studies, however, in our everyday life chronic sleep deficiency is more common than 24–48 hours of sleep deprivation. People generally sleep longer on weekends than workdays. For instance, a recent survey shows that nurses get on average 84 minutes more sleep on non-work days than workdays. This suggests that people are not getting enough sleep on workdays and trying to "catch up" on weekends. It has been reported that people's performance on testing of attention and serial mathematical calculations under one week of sleep restriction to five hours of sleep per night is as poor as that under 24 hours of total sleep loss. This suggests that sleep loss is cumulative. By the end of the workweek, the sleep debt is significant enough to impair people's learning and decision-making during work or everyday life. A 2016 survey published by the *McKinsey Quarterly* shows that 46% of business leaders believe that lack of sleep has little impact on their leadership performance. 43% of the leaders do not get enough sleep at least four nights a week. Now is the time for the leaders to update their viewpoint and get enough sleep.

In his bestselling book *Dreamland: Adventures in the Strange Science of Sleep*, David K. Randall told the story that the U.S. Defense Advanced Research Projects Agency spent millions of dollars trying to find a way for soldiers to go without sleep for one hundred hours and still perform common tasks normally. Yet, none of their tests worked. "No drug or procedure has been found to replicate and replace the benefits of sleep. It is unlikely that there ever will be," Randall wrote. "The only way to recover from lost sleep was to get more of it later."

How much sleep is enough for us to maintain everyday optimal functioning? Generally, adults need 7–9 hours of sleep per day to sustain optimum alertness and maintain optimal functioning. Obtaining enough sleep day-to-day is important, but obtaining high-quality sleep is essential as well. Several specific strategies that help to optimize each sleep opportunity are presented below:

1) Establish more regularity and consistency in the timing of daily activities, especially the timing of getting up, evening meals, and bedtime routine. For instance, you may form a habit of reading, taking a hot shower, and then going to bed. Higher levels of regularity in behavioral rhythms are associated with better sleep outcomes, lower depression, and improved health.

2) Do not use light-emitting electronic devices such as cellphone and tablets before bedtime, as these devices exert negative effects on sleep.

3) Try to reduce the total sitting time and television viewing while sitting. Each extra hour per day of total sitting is associated with higher odds of poor sleep quality. Each extra hour per day of television viewing while sitting is associated with greater odds of long sleep onset latency ($\geq$ 30 minutes), waking up too early in the morning, poor sleep quality, and high risk for obstructive sleep apnea.

4) Perform aerobic exercise every day. But try to avoid vigorous exercise two hours before going to bed, as vigorous late-night exercise may produce increased arousal and lead to longer sleep onset latency.

Regular exercise makes you sleep more soundly. Dozens of studies have shown that people who exercise regularly, for instance walking, running, cycling, doing Taichi, and so on, find it easier to fall asleep, have fewer awakenings at night, and feel more rested in the morning. They also feel less sleepy and more energetic throughout the day. This is true whether you are young or old, and whether you have or do not have sleep problems.

Exercise and sleep well.

12. Exercise Helps Executives Beat Jet Lag

I do not suffer from jet lag, only with difficulties in sleeping.

— An Olympic athlete after flying from the U.K. to Australia

In 1997, Bernhard Liese, Director of the Health Services Department of the World Bank, published a report on the medical insurance claims by its over 10,000 staff and consultants. These claims include infectious diseases, back disorders, injuries, and psychological disorders. Liese found a surprising pattern: those who traveled internationally had a higher rate of insurance claims than those who did not. The more the international trips, the more the insurance claims. For instance, compared to those without international travel, men who traveled once, 2–3 times, and over four times report 1.28-, 1.54-, and 1.97-fold increase in insurance claims for infectious diseases. The claims were more increased for psychological disorders. Compared to those without international travel, men who traveled once, 2–3 times, and over four times report 2.11-, 3.13-, and 3.06-fold increase in insurance claims for psychological disorders. This report drew lots of attention to the problems related to international business travel. Researchers eventually recognized that it is not the international travel per se, but the "jet lag" caused by international travel that was to be blamed.

Jet lag is a syndrome caused by a disruption of the body clock due to rapid changes in the light and dark cycle. It is associated with many psychological and physical problems, including impaired alertness, daytime fatigue, disturbance in sleep, anxiety, depression, irritability, gastrointestinal problems, and malaise.

Jet lag also compromises work performance. After analyzing decades of data involving tens of thousands of games, researchers found that jet lag impaired professional sports performance in baseball, football, and basketball players. In a paper titled "Baseball Teams Beaten By Jet Lag" published in the journal *Nature*, Lawrence Recht at the University of Massachusetts analyzed three complete season records of the North American Major League Baseball games based on whether there was transcontinental traveling or not. Recht found that irrespective of the true competence of the teams, the winning rate of the home team was about 54.1% when the other team did not travel. When the other team did westward traveling, the winning rate of the home team increased to 56.2%.

Furthermore, when the other team did eastward traveling, the winning rate of the home team increased to 62.9%. These results could not be explained by a "home field" advantage because the home field advantage was the same across the three situations. It shows that jet lag decreases the visiting teams' performance.

The incidence and severity of jet lag increase with the number of time zones crossed. It affects most travelers crossing five or more time zones. Furthermore, the influence is higher for eastward than westward traveling.

Millions of people travel around the world and across time zones each year for business and holidays. We would expect the influences of jet lag to be substantial. Unfortunately, due to a lack of research, right now scientists can only offer limited recommendations:

1) Try to get an adequate amount of sleep before travel.

2) Be prepared for changes in sleep pattern.

3) Upon arrival, take appropriate naps.

4) Take medicine.

A piece of good news is that exercise is also effective in helping travelers to adapt to new time zones and beat jet lag.

In November 2016, I went to San Diego to attend the annual scientific meeting of Society for Neuroscience. On the flight from Tokyo to Los Angeles (local time in Los Angeles is 17 hours behind Tokyo), I came across a paper published 20 years ago by M Shiota at Yamaguchi University in Japan. Shiota studied ten airline crewmembers flying from Tokyo to Los Angeles (what a coincidence!). On the day following arrival at Los Angeles (Day 3), Shiota asked half of the crewmembers to exercise outdoors for about five hours and the other half to remain in their room or go shopping. Shiota found that on Day 4, the crewmembers who exercised showed biological measures indicating better adaptation to the new local time zone.

Yujiro Yamanaka at Hokkaido University in Japan recently replicated the finding. Yamanaka asked subjects to spend 12 days in a temporal isolation facility with dim lighting conditions and phase-advanced their sleep schedule by eight hours from their habitual sleep times for four days. This is equivalent to asking them to travel eastward crossing eight time zones, which causes serious jet lag. After that, during the next six consecutive days, Yamanaka removed all time cues from the subjects. As the experimental manipulation, he asked half of the subjects to run with a bicycle ergometer in the morning and at noon of the new schedule for two hours each day. In contrast, he asked the other half of the subjects to sit on a chair during those times. It turned out that during these days, those in the exercise group found it much easier to adapt to the new schedule. They were able to fall asleep easily and sleep better. Exercise promotes the resynchronization to a new environment of the circadian rhythm.

Upon arriving at a new destination for business or leisure, try to exercise every day. It will help you adapt to the new time zone and work effectively.

POSTSCRIPT

In a 1988 study, David Frew and Nealia Bruning in the U.S. reported that commercial real estate stock brokers who attended a 12-week-long aerobic exercise program had higher sales during and after the program as opposed to their colleagues who didn't attend. In a 2005 study, Jim McKenna at Leeds Metropolitan University in the U.K. reported that on days when workers exercised, their time management skills, mental performance and ability to meet deadlines increased. Overall, exercise led to a boost in job performance by approximately 15%. In a 2009 meta-analysis of 138 studies published between 1969 and 2007 involving over 38,000 subjects, Vicki S. Conn at the University of Missouri in the U.S. concluded that workplace exercise programs reduce job stress, and increase work attendance and job satisfaction. These findings reinforce the idea that exercise is a potent strategy for improving work performance.

As we have shown throughout this book, exercise can be flexibly used in everyday life to boost performance. Regular exercise builds your fitness and brain efficiency, which is a highway towards productivity, leadership and excellence. Fitness is personal capital, which gains you an advantage to benefit more from exercise. Furthermore, exercising alone improves your own productivity and leadership skills. Exercising with your employee or superior brings a win-win situation to both of you. Exercising with your family brings three degrees of benefits.

But exercising alone is far from enough for high performance and great leadership. As suggested by many renowned developmental psychologists, our lives are the sum of all our life experiences. Similarly, your productivity and leadership is the sum of all the effective strategies you have learned from your own experiences and other sources. To become a high-performing leader, you need more strategies. The Japanese translator of this book, Dr. Yasuhiro Mochizuki, is a meditator. Mochizuki once shared with me his experience of "seeing the surrounding views more clearly" after each weekly waterfall meditation. Meditation is a practice used to develop a state of mindfulness. The benefit of mindfulness and meditation on the mind and brain has also received scientific support. It may be another effective strategy to boost productivity and improve leadership.

If you want to learn more strategies, please feel free to sign up for my newsletter through

http://brainandlife.net. If you enjoyed this book, please leave a brief review on Amazon or Goodreads. Thanks.

Enjoy exercise and explore more. Are you ready to challenge your potential?

ACKNOWLEDGEMENTS

Many people provided helpful comments and suggestions for this book. Si Yang, Takaaki Yuzawa, Heather Saxton, Yasuhiro Mochizuki, Hermione Bloom, Cate Courtright, and Hua Shi, thank you. All of you have provided insightful ideas—although none is responsible for any errors in this book. I also thank my book cover designer Hongtao Chen for giving me a pool of wonderful options, although I like this one the best.

I am grateful to my editor Ray Dawn for her professional advice and assistance in polishing this book. Ray helped me realize my own writing habits and tried to teach me how to write proper English with the book as a practical example. Ray, thank you so much.

I'd like to express my gratitude to Jean Paul Zogby for his invaluable help during the launch of the book. Jean Paul, thank you. I also thank Russell Burgess and Matija Kolaric for their help.

REFERENCES

PREFACE

A survey of the top 3,000... Neck, C. P., & Cooper, K. H.
(2000). The fit executive: Exercise and diet guidelines for
enhancing performance. *The Academy of Management
Executive*, 14(2), 72-83; Neck, C. P., Mitchell, T. L., Manz, C.
C., & Thompson, E. C. (2004). *Fit to lead: The proven 8-week
solution for shaping up your body, your mind, and your career*.
Macmillan.

In many countries... World Health Organization (2010).
Global status report on noncommunicable diseases 2010.
World Health 176 (2010). doi:978 92 4 156422 9; Centers for
Disease Control. (2010). Healthy People 2010 final review;
Kohl III, H. W., & Cook, H. D. (Eds.). (2013). *Educating the
student body: Taking physical activity and physical education
to school*. National Academies Press; Sallis, J. F., Bull, F.,
Guthold, R., Heath, G. W., Inoue, S., Kelly, P.,... & Lancet
Physical Activity Series 2 Executive Committee. (2016).
Progress in physical activity over the Olympic quadrennium.
The Lancet, *388*(10051), 1325-1336; Liu, Y. (2017).
Promoting physical activity among Chinese youth: No time to
wait. *Journal of Sport and Health Science*.

CHAPTER 1

For the details of the Harvard Grant Study... Vaillant, G. E.
(1977). Adaptation to life. Harvard University Press; Vaillant,
G. E. (2012). *Triumphs of experience*. Harvard University

Press; Joshua Wolf Shenk. (JUNE 2009). What Makes Us Happy? *The Atlantic. Available* https://www.theatlantic.com/magazine/archive/2009/06/what-makes-us-happy/307439/ finally accessed 2017.04.24

CHAPTER 2

Our working memory is limited... Conway, A. R., Kane, M. J., & Engle, R. W. (2003). Working memory capacity and its relation to general intelligence. *Trends in cognitive sciences, 7*(12), 547-552.

Cognitive flexibility... Dajani, D. R., & Uddin, L. Q. (2015). Demystifying cognitive flexibility: Implications for clinical and developmental neuroscience. *Trends in neurosciences, 38*(9), 571-578.

Physically fit people have higher executive functions... Bunce, D. J., Barrowclough, A., & Morris, I. (1996). The moderating influence of physical fitness on age gradients in vigilance and serial choice responding tasks. *Psychology and aging,* 11(4), 671; Kao, S. C., Westfall, D. R., Parks, A. C., Pontifex, M. B., & Hillman, C. H. (2016). Muscular and Aerobic Fitness, Working Memory, and Academic Achievement in Children. *Medicine and Science in Sports and Exercise*; Ishihara, T., Sugasawa, S., Matsuda, Y., & Mizuno, M. (2017). Relationship between sports experience and executive function in 6–12-year-old children: independence from physical fitness and moderation by gender. *Developmental Science.*

Fit postal workers... Frew, D. R., & Bruning, N. S. (1988). Improved Productivity and Job Satisfaction Through Employee. *Hospital Materiel Management Quarterly*, 9(4), 62.

Fit corporate employees... Pronk, N. P., Martinson, B., Kessler, R. C., Beck, A. L., Simon, G. E., & Wang, P. (2004). The association between work performance and physical activity, cardiorespiratory fitness, and obesity. *Journal of Occupational and Environmental Medicine*, 46(1), 19-25.

FMRI to study the brain... Chaddock-Heyman, L., Erickson, K. I., Voss, M., Knecht, A., Pontifex, M. B., Castelli, D.,... & Kramer, A. (2013). The effects of physical activity on functional MRI activation associated with cognitive control in children: a randomized controlled intervention. *Frontiers in human neuroscience*, 7, 72.

People with higher IQs... Neubauer, A. C., & Fink, A. (2009). Intelligence and neural efficiency. *Neuroscience & Biobehavioral Reviews*, 33(7), 1004-1023.

CHAPTER 3

For the details of adult neurogenesis... Deng, W., Aimone, J. B., & Gage, F. H. (2010). New neurons and new memories: how does adult hippocampal neurogenesis affect learning and memory?. *Nature Reviews Neuroscience*, 11(5), 339-350; Opendak, M., & Gould, E. (2015). Adult neurogenesis: a substrate for experience-dependent change. *Trends in cognitive sciences*, 19(3), 151-161.

cerebral blood volume... Palmer, T. D., Willhoite, A. R., & Gage, F. H. (2000). Vascular niche for adult hippocampal neurogenesis. *Journal of Comparative Neurology, 425*(4), 479-494.

endurance is positively associated... Burdette, J. H., Laurienti, P. J., Espeland, M. A., Morgan, A. R., Telesford, Q., Vechlekar, C. D.,... & Rejeski, W. J. (2010). Using network science to evaluate exercise-associated brain changes in older adults. *Frontiers in aging neuroscience, 2*, 23; Chaddock-Heyman, L., Erickson, K. I., Chappell, M. A., Johnson, C. L., Kienzler, C., Knecht, A.,... & Hillman, C. H. (2016). Aerobic fitness is associated with greater hippocampal cerebral blood flow in children. *Developmental Cognitive Neuroscience, 20*, 52-58; Maass, A., Düzel, S., Goerke, M., Becke, A., Sobieray, U., Neumann, K.,... & Ahrens, D. (2015). Vascular hippocampal plasticity after aerobic exercise in older adults. *Molecular psychiatry, 20*(5), 585-593; Heo, S., Prakash, R. S., Voss, M. W., Erickson, K. I., Ouyang, C., Sutton, B. P., & Kramer, A. F. (2010). Resting hippocampal blood flow, spatial memory and aging. *Brain research, 1315*, 119-127.

a 12-week aerobic fitness... Pereira, A. C., Huddleston, D. E., Brickman, A. M., Sosunov, A. A., Hen, R., McKhann, G. M.,... & Small, S. A. (2007). An in vivo correlate of exercise-induced neurogenesis in the adult dentate gyrus. *Proceedings of the National Academy of Sciences, 104*(13), 5638-5643.

CHAPTER 4

For the details of stress response… Sapolsky, R. M. (2004). Why zebras don't get ulcers: The acclaimed guide to stress, stress-related diseases, and coping-now revised and updated. Macmillan.

Fit people have higher stress tolerance…Boullosa, D. A., Hautala, A. J., & Leicht, A. S. (2014). Introduction to the research topic: the role of physical fitness on cardiovascular responses to stress. Frontiers in physiology, 5; Rodrigues, A. V. S., Martinez, E. C., Duarte, A. F. A., & Ribeiro, L. C. S. (2007). Aerobic fitness and its influence in the mental stress response in army personnel. Revista Brasileira de Medicina do Esporte, 13(2), 113-117.

CHAPTER 5

Two keys for building… Neck, C. P., Mitchell, T. L., Manz, C. C., & Thompson, E. C. (2004). *Fit to lead: The proven 8-week solution for shaping up your body, your mind, and your career.* Macmillan.

Fitness drops about 30-50%... Daley, M. J., & Spinks, W. L. (2000). Exercise, mobility and aging. *Sports Medicine*, *29*(1), 1-12.

BDNF… Szuhany, K. L., Bugatti, M., & Otto, M. W. (2015). A meta-analytic review of the effects of exercise on brain-derived neurotrophic factor. *Journal of psychiatric research*, *60*, 56-64.

IGF-1... Borst, S. E., De Hoyos, D. V., Garzarella, L. I. N. D. A., Vincent, K. E. V. I. N., Pollock, B. H., Lowenthal, D. T., & Pollock, M. L. (2001). Effects of resistance training on insulin-like growth factor-I and IGF binding proteins. *Medicine and science in sports and exercise*, 33(4), 648-653.

For adults by the WHO... World Health Organization (2010). W. H. O. Global recommendations on physical activity for health. Geneva: World Health Organization (2010). doi:10.1080/11026480410034349

At least 20 minutes of resistance exercise... Neck, C. P., Mitchell, T. L., Manz, C. C., & Thompson, E. C. (2004). *Fit to lead: The proven 8-week solution for shaping up your body, your mind, and your career*. Macmillan.

High saturated fat diet... Dingess, P. M., Darling, R. A., Dolence, E. K., Culver, B. W., & Brown, T. E. (2016). Exposure to a diet high in fat attenuates dendritic spine density in the medial prefrontal cortex. *Brain Structure and Function*, 1-9; Lavagnino, L., Arnone, D., Cao, B., Soares, J. C., & Selvaraj, S. (2016). Inhibitory control in obesity and binge eating disorder: A systematic review and meta-analysis of neurocognitive and neuroimaging studies. *Neuroscience & Biobehavioral Reviews*, 68, 714-726; Luppino, F. S., de Wit, L. M., Bouvy, P. F., Stijnen, T., Cuijpers, P., Penninx, B. W., & Zitman, F. G. (2010). Overweight, obesity, and depression: a systematic review and meta-analysis of longitudinal studies. Archives of general psychiatry, 67(3), 220-229; Heberden, C. (2016). Modulating adult neurogenesis through dietary interventions. *Nutrition Research Reviews*, 1-9.

The Mediterranean-style diet… Sofi, F., Abbate, R., Gensini, G. F., & Casini, A. (2010). Accruing evidence on benefits of adherence to the Mediterranean diet on health: an updated systematic review and meta-analysis. *The American journal of clinical nutrition*, *92*(5), 1189-1196; Lourida, I., Soni, M., Thompson-Coon, J., Purandare, N., Lang, I. A., Ukoumunne, O. C., & Llewellyn, D. J. (2013). Mediterranean diet, cognitive function, and dementia: a systematic review. *Epidemiology*, *24*(4), 479-489; Tran, L. V., Malla, B. A., Sharma, A. N., Kumar, S., Tyagi, N., & Tyagi, A. K. (2016). Effect of omega-3 and omega-6 polyunsaturated fatty acid enriched diet on plasma IGF-1 and testosterone concentration, puberty and semen quality in male buffalo. *Animal Reproduction Science*, 173, 63-72.

CHAPTER 6

Charles Darwin… Darwin, C. (1958). *The Autobiography of Charles Darwin*, ed. Nora Barlow.

Michael Mangum… Neck, C. P., Mitchell, T. L., Manz, C. C., & Thompson, E. C. (2004). *Fit to lead: The proven 8-week solution for shaping up your body, your mind, and your career.* Macmillan.

Two psychologists at Stanford… Oppezzo, M., & Schwartz, D. L. (2014). Give your ideas some legs: The positive effect of walking on creative thinking. *Journal of experimental psychology: learning, memory, and cognition*, 40(4), 1142.

Hannah Steinberg at Middlesex… Steinberg, H., Sykes, E. A., Moss, T., Lowery, S., LeBoutillier, N., & Dewey, A. (1997).

Exercise enhances creativity independently of mood. *British Journal of Sports Medicine*, 31(3), 240-245.

CHAPTER 7

Robert Thayer at California... Thayer, R. E., Newman, J. R., & McClain, T. M. (1994). Self-regulation of mood: Strategies for changing a bad mood, raising energy, and reducing tension. *Journal of personality and social psychology*, *67*(5), 910.

Maxime Taquet at Harvard... Taquet, M., Quoidbach, J., de Montjoye, Y. A., Desseilles, M., & Gross, J. J. (2016). Hedonism and the choice of everyday activities. *Proceedings of the National Academy of Sciences*, 201519998.

brisk walking for only ten... Thayer, R. E. (1987). Problem perception, optimism, and related states as a function of time of day (diurnal rhythm) and moderate exercise: Two arousal systems in interaction. *Motivation and Emotion*, *11*(1), 19-36; Thayer, R. E. (1987). Energy, tiredness, and tension effects of a sugar snack versus moderate exercise. *Journal of personality and social psychology*, *52*(1), 119; Thayer, R. E., Peters, D. P., Takahashi, P. J., & Birkhead-Flight, A. M. (1993). Mood and behavior (smoking and sugar snacking) following moderate exercise: A partial test of self-regulation theory. *Personality and Individual Differences*, *14*(1), 97-104.

hundreds of studies... Petruzzello, S. J., Landers, D. M., Hatfield, B. D., Kubitz, K. A., & Salazar, W. (1991). A meta-analysis on the anxiety-reducing effects of acute and chronic exercise. *Sports medicine*, *11*(3), 143-182; Hamer, M., Taylor, A., & Steptoe, A. (2006). The effect of acute aerobic exercise on stress related blood pressure responses: a systematic review and meta-analysis. *Biological psychology*, *71*(2), 183-190; Reed, J., & Ones, D. S. (2006). The effect of acute aerobic exercise on positive activated affect: A meta-analysis. *Psychology of Sport and Exercise*, *7*(5), 477-514.

CHAPTER 8

Executives burnout... Levinson, H. (1996 July-August). When executives burn out. *Harvard business review*, 153-63

30% of teachers and... Linden, D. V. D., Keijsers, G. P., Eling, P., & Schaijk, R. V. (2005). Work stress and attentional difficulties: An initial study on burnout and cognitive failures. *Work & Stress*, *19*(1), 23-36; Unterbrink, T., Hack, A., Pfeifer, R., Buhl-Grießhaber, V., Müller, U., Wesche, H.,... & Bauer, J. (2007). Burnout and effort–reward-imbalance in a sample of 949 German teachers. *International archives of occupational and environmental health*, *80*(5), 433-441

96% of senior leaders... Kwoh, L. (2013). When the CEO Burns Out: Job Fatigue Catches up to Some Executive Amid Mounting Expectations; No More Forced Smiles. *The Wall Street Journal*, May 8

Hidehiko Takahashi at Kyoto... Tei, S., Becker, C., Kawada, R., Fujino, J., Jankowski, K. F., Sugihara, G.,... & Takahashi, H. (2014). Can we predict burnout severity from empathy-related brain activity?. *Translational psychiatry*, 4(6), e393.

72% of executives... Creative Staffing Group. (2015). THE ALLURE OF ENDLESS SUMMERS: Managers and Workers

See an Upside to an Unlimited Vacation Policy, But Most Wouldn't Take Advantage of the Perk. http://creativegroup.mediaroom.com/unlimited-vacation

Magnus Lindwall at the University of Gothenburg... Lindwall, M., Gerber, M., Jonsdottir, I. H., Börjesson, M., & Ahlborg Jr, G. (2014). The relationships of change in physical activity with change in depression, anxiety, and burnout: A longitudinal study of Swedish healthcare workers. *Health Psychology*, *33*(11), 1309.

Timothy Puetz at University of Georgia... Puetz, T. W., O'connor, P. J., & Dishman, R. K. (2006). Effects of chronic exercise on feelings of energy and fatigue: a quantitative synthesis. *Psychological bulletin*, *132*(6), 866.

Reduces the risk of burnout by 62%... Olson, S. M., Odo, N. U., Duran, A. M., Pereira, A. G., & Mandel, J. H. (2014). Burnout and physical activity in Minnesota internal medicine resident physicians. *Journal of graduate medical education*, 6(4), 669-674.

CHAPTER 9

Impairs workplace performance... Wang, M. L., & Tsai, L. J. (2014). Work–Family conflict and job performance in nurses: The moderating effects of social support. *Journal of Nursing Research*, 22(3), 200-207; Kan, D., & Yu, X. (2016). Occupational stress, work-family conflict and depressive symptoms among Chinese bank employees: The role of psychological capital. *International journal of environmental research and public health*, 13(1), 134.

Morgan Krannitz at The Pennsylvania State University... Krannitz, M. A., Grandey, A. A., Liu, S., & Almeida, D. A. (2015). Workplace surface acting and marital partner discontent: Anxiety and exhaustion spillover mechanisms.

Josje Dikkers at Radboud University Nijmegen... Dikkers, J. S., Geurts, S. A., Kinnunen, U., Kompier, M. A., & Taris, T. W. (2007). Crossover between work and home in dyadic partner relationships. *Scandinavian Journal of Psychology*, *48*(6), 529-538.

Eva Roos at University of Helsinki... Roos, E., Sarlio-Lähteenkorva, S., Lallukka, T., & Lahelma, E. (2007). Associations of work–family conflicts with food habits and physical activity. *Public health nutrition*, 10(03), 222-229.

David M. Almeida at The Pennsylvania State University... Lee, B., Lawson, K. M., Chang, P. J., Neuendorf, C., Dmitrieva, N. O., & Almeida, D. M. (2015). Leisure-time physical activity moderates the longitudinal associations between work-family spillover and physical health. *Journal of leisure research*, 47(4).

Children in families with more work-family conflict... Erel, O., & Burman, B. (1995). Interrelatedness of marital relations and parent-child relations: a meta-analytic review. *Psychological bulletin*, 118(1), 108; Kamp Dush, C. M., & Taylor, M. G. (2012). Trajectories of marital conflict across the life course: Predictors and interactions with marital happiness trajectories. *Journal of family issues*, 33(3), 341-368.

CHAPTER 10

Positive emotions make us achieve more... Lyubomirsky, S., King, L., & Diener, E. (2005). The benefits of frequent positive affect: Does happiness lead to success?.

Positive emotions not only feel good... Fredrickson, B. L. (2013). Positive emotions broaden and build. In E. Ashby Plant & P.G. Devine (Eds.), *Advances on Experimental Social Psychology*, 47, 1-53. Burlington: Academic Press.

Harvard management scientist Teresa Amabile... Amabile, T., & Kramer, S. (2011). The progress principle. *Harvard Business Review Press, Boston, MA*.

Neuroscientific research has shown... Aron, A., Fisher, H., Mashek, D. J., Strong, G., Li, H., & Brown, L. L. (2005). Reward, motivation, and emotion systems associated with early-stage intense romantic love. *Journal of neurophysiology*, *94*(1), 327-337; Rademacher, L., Krach, S., Kohls, G., Irmak, A., Gründer, G., & Spreckelmeyer, K. N. (2010). Dissociation of neural networks for anticipation and consumption of monetary and social rewards. *Neuroimage*, *49*(4), 3276-3285; Lin, A., Adolphs, R., & Rangel, A. (2012). Social and monetary reward learning engage overlapping neural substrates. *Social cognitive and affective neuroscience*, *7*(3), 274-281; Montague, P. R., King-Casas, B., & Cohen, J. D. (2006). Imaging valuation models in human choice. *Annu. Rev. Neurosci.*, *29*, 417-448; Ruff, C. C., & Fehr, E. (2014). The neurobiology of rewards and values in social decision making. *Nature Reviews Neuroscience*, *15*(8), 549-562; Bartels, A., &

Zeki, S. (2004). The neural correlates of maternal and romantic love. *Neuroimage, 21*(3), 1155-1166.

Robert Thayer at California State University... Thayer, R. E. (1987). Problem perception, optimism, and related states as a function of time of day (diurnal rhythm) and moderate exercise: Two arousal systems in interaction. *Motivation and Emotion, 11*(1), 19-36; Thayer, R. E. (1987). Energy, tiredness, and tension effects of a sugar snack versus moderate exercise. *Journal of personality and social psychology, 52*(1), 119; Thayer, R. E., Peters, D. P., Takahashi, P. J., & Birkhead-Flight, A. M. (1993). Mood and behavior (smoking and sugar snacking) following moderate exercise: A partial test of self-regulation theory. *Personality and Individual Differences, 14*(1), 97-104.

Cheryl J. Hansen at Northern Arizona University ... Hansen, C. J., Stevens, L. C., & Coast, J. R. (2001). Exercise duration and mood state: How much is enough to feel better?. *Health Psychology, 20*(4), 267-275.

CHAPTER 11

Two professors at Loughborough University... Harrison, Y., & Horne, J. A. (1999). One night of sleep loss impairs innovative thinking and flexible decision making. *Organizational behavior and human decision processes, 78*(2), 128-145.

Julian Lim and David Dinges at the University of Pennsylvania... Lim, J., & Dinges, D. F. (2010). A meta-analysis of the impact of short-term sleep deprivation on cognitive variables.

Nurses get on average... Caldwell, J. A., Mallis, M. M., Caldwell, J. L., Paul, M. A., Miller, J. C., & Neri, D. F. (2009). Fatigue countermeasures in aviation. *Aviation, space, and environmental medicine, 80*(1), 29-59.

One week of sleep restriction to 5 hours... Linde, L., & Bergströme, M. (1992). The effect of one night without sleep on problem-solving and immediate recall. *Psychological research, 54*(2), 127-136; Polzella, D. J. (1975). Effects of sleep deprivation on short-term recognition memory. *Journal of Experimental Psychology: Human Learning and Memory, 1*(2), 194; Jewett, M. E., Dijk, D. J., Kronauer, R. E., & Dinges, D. F. (1999). Dose-response relationship between sleep duration and human psychomotor vigilance and subjective alertness. *Sleep: Journal of Sleep Research & Sleep Medicine.*

46% of business leaders... van Dam, N., & van der Helm, E. (2016). The organizational cost of insufficient sleep. *McKinsey Quarterly, February 2016.*

In his bestselling book... Randall, D. K. (2012). Dreamland: Adventures in the strange science of sleep. WW Norton & Company.

Adults need 7-9 hours of sleep... Hirshkowitz, M., Whiton, K., Albert, S. M., Alessi, C., Bruni, O., DonCarlos, L.,... & Kheirandish-Gozal, L. (2015). National Sleep Foundation's updated sleep duration recommendations: final report. *Sleep Health,* 1(4), 233-243.

Several specific strategies... Caldwell, J. A., Mallis, M. M., Caldwell, J. L., Paul, M. A., Miller, J. C., & Neri, D. F. (2009). Fatigue countermeasures in aviation. *Aviation, space, and environmental medicine, 80*(1), 29-59; MYLLYMÄKI, T., KYRÖLÄINEN, H., Savolainen, K., Hokka, L., Jakonen, R., Juuti, T., MARTINMÄKI, K., Kaartinen, J., KINNUNEN, M.L. and Rusko, H. (2011). Effects of vigorous late-night exercise on sleep quality and cardiac autonomic activity. *Journal of sleep research*, 20(1pt2), 146-153; Dautovich, N.D., Shoji, K.D. and McCrae, C.S. (2013). Variety is the Spice of Life: A Microlongitudinal Study Examining Age Differences in Intraindividual Variability in Daily Activities in Relation to Sleep Outcomes. *The Journals of Gerontology Series B: Psychological Sciences and Social Sciences*, p.gbt120; Chang, A. M., Aeschbach, D., Duffy, J. F., & Czeisler, C. A. (2015). Evening use of light-emitting eReaders negatively affects sleep, circadian timing, and next-morning alertness. *Proceedings of the National Academy of Sciences*, 112(4), 1232-1237; Buman, M.P., Kline, C.E., Youngstedt, S.D., Phillips, B., de Mello, M.T. and Hirshkowitz, M. (2015). Sitting and television viewing: novel risk factors for sleep disturbance and apnea risk? Results from the 2013 national sleep foundation sleep in america poll. *CHEST Journal*, 147(3), 728-734.

Regular exercise makes you sleep... Kredlow, M.A., Capozzoli, M.C., Hearon, B.A., Calkins, A.W. and Otto, M.W. (2015). The effects of physical activity on sleep: a meta-analytic review. *Journal of behavioral medicine*, 38(3), 427-449; Lang, C., Kalak, N., Brand, S., Holsboer-Trachsler, E.,

Pühse, U. and Gerber, M. (2016). The relationship between physical activity and sleep from mid adolescence to early adulthood. A systematic review of methodological approaches and meta-analysis. *Sleep medicine reviews*, 28, 28-41; Yang, P.Y., Ho, K.H., Chen, H.C. and Chien, M.Y. (2012). Exercise training improves sleep quality in middle-aged and older adults with sleep problems: a systematic review. *Journal of physiotherapy*, 58(3), 157-163; Du, S., Dong, J., Zhang, H., Jin, S., Xu, G., Liu, Z., Chen, L., Yin, H. and Sun, Z. (2015). Taichi exercise for self-rated sleep quality in older people: A systematic review and meta-analysis. *International journal of nursing studies*, 52(1), 368-379.

CHAPTER 12

Bernhard Liese, Director of... Liese, B., Mundt, K. A., Dell, L. D., Nagy, L., & Demure, B. (1997). Medical insurance claims associated with international business travel. *Occupational and Environmental Medicine*, 54(7), 499-503.

For details of jet lag... Waterhouse, J., Reilly, T., Atkinson, G., & Edwards, B. (2007). Jet lag: trends and coping strategies. *The Lancet*, 369(9567), 1117-1129; Sack, R. L. (2010). Jet lag. *New England Journal of Medicine*, 362(5), 440-447; Song, A., Severini, T., & Allada, R. (2017). How jet lag impairs Major League Baseball performance. *Proceedings of the National Academy of Sciences*, 114(6), 1407-1412; Herxheimer, A. (2014). Jet lag. *BMJ clinical evidence*, 2014.

Jet lag also compromises work performance... Striker, J., Dimberg, L., & Liese, B. H. (2000). Stress and business travel:

Individual, managerial, and corporate concerns. *Global Business and Organizational Excellence*, 20(1), 3-10.

jet lag impairs professional sports… Steenland, K., & Deddens, J. A. (1997). Effect of travel and rest on performance of professional basketball players. *Sleep*, 20(5), 366-369; Recht, L. D., Lew, R. A., & Schwartz, W. J. (1995). Baseball teams beaten by jet lag. *Nature*, 377(6550), 583-583.

M Shiota at Yamaguchi University… Shiota, M., Sudou, M. and Ohshima, M. (1996). Using outdoor exercise to decrease jet lag in airline crewmembers. *Aviation, space, and environmental medicine*, 67(12), 1155-1160.

Yujiro Yamanaka at Hokkaido University… Yamanaka, Y., Hashimoto, S., Tanahashi, Y., Nishide, S.Y., Honma, S. and Honma, K.I. (2010). Physical exercise accelerates reentrainment of human sleep-wake cycle but not of plasma melatonin rhythm to 8-h phase-advanced sleep schedule. *American Journal of Physiology-Regulatory, Integrative and Comparative Physiology*, 298(3), R681-R691.

POSTSCRIPT

David Frew and Nealia Bruning in the U.S…. Frew, D. R., & Bruning, N. S. (1988). Improved Productivity and Job Satisfaction Through Employee. *Hospital materiel management quarterly*, 9(4), 62.

Jim McKenna at Leeds Metropolitan University… Coulson, J. C., McKenna, J., & Field, M. (2008). Exercising at work and self-reported work performance. *International Journal of Workplace Health Management, 1*(3), 176-197.

Vicki S. Conn at the University of Missouri… Conn, V. S., Hafdahl, A. R., Cooper, P. S., Brown, L. M., & Lusk, S. L. (2009). Meta-analysis of workplace physical activity interventions. *American journal of preventive medicine, 37*(4), 330-339.

ABOUT THE AUTHOR

Dr. Chong Chen is a neuroscientist and possesses a Ph.D. in Medicine. Chong has authored 10 books, including two series called **The Anchor of Our Purest Thoughts** and **Your Baby's Developing Brain**.

As far as the future goes, Chong hopes that he will be able to translate scientific findings into ways that will allow regular people to live better lives. And through his books, he hopes that he can reach a much wider audience.

You can contact Chong and follow what he is writing about at: https://brainandlife.net.